KETO CHAFFLE

LOSE WEIGHT BY STIMULATING THE BRAIN AND
METABOLISM: DELICIUS RECIPES LOW CARB TO
INTEGRATE YOUR KETOGENIC DIET

CHRISTINE BUCKLEY

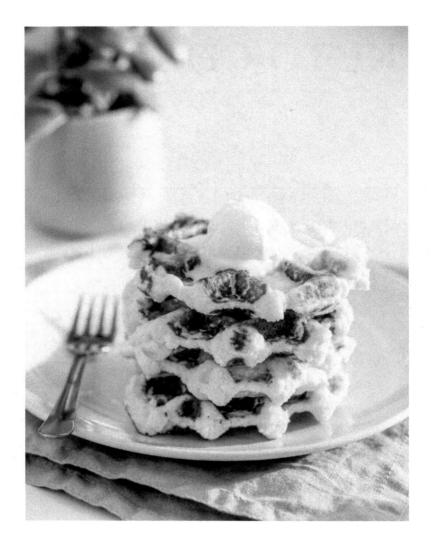

The following Book is reproduced below with the goal of providing information that is as accurate and reliable as possible. Regardless, purchasing this Book can be seen as consent to the fact that both the publisher and the author of this book are in no way experts on the topics discussed within and that any recommendations or suggestions that are made herein are for entertainment purposes only. Professionals should be consulted as needed prior to undertaking any of the action endorsed herein.

This declaration is deemed fair and valid by both the American Bar Association and the Committee of Publishers Association and is legally binding throughout the United States.

Furthermore, the transmission, duplication, or reproduction of any of the following work including specific information will be considered an illegal act irrespective of if it is done electronically or in print. This extends to creating a secondary or tertiary copy of the work or a recorded copy and is only allowed with the express written consent from the Publisher. All additional right reserved.

The information in the following pages is broadly considered a truthful and accurate account of facts and as such, any inattention, use, or misuse of the information in question by the reader will render any resulting actions solely under their purview. There are no scenarios in which the publisher or the original author of this work can be in any fashion deemed liable for any hardship or damages that may befall them after undertaking information described herein.

Additionally, the information in the following pages is intended only for informational purposes and should thus be thought of as universal. As befitting its nature, it is presented without assurance regarding its prolonged validity or interim quality. Trademarks that are mentioned are done without written consent and can in no way be considered an endorsement from the trademark holder.

TABLE OF CONTENTS

INTRODUCTION

Keto chaffles have taken the world by storm. Made with just two main ingredients, egg and butter, they can be prepared easily at home. You can eat them as sweet desserts, as a breakfast food, or as a snack. Chaffles are perfectly healthy foods that follow the ketogenic diet recommendations.

They are high-fat, protein, and low-carbohydrate foods that can show the body how to use fat as an alternative source of fuel to produce energy and burn fat.

Thank you for downloading this book.

In this book, I will discuss chaffles and explain how they are different than waffles. I will ex- plain the various types of chaffles you can make easily at home. I will also go deep into the ketogenic diet and discuss its many advantages.

Finally, I will also share many mouth-watering Keto Chaffle recipes that are all easy to prepare. For each recipe, I will provide a list of ingredients and detailed step-by-step instructions. I am sure you will find this book very useful. Happy reading!

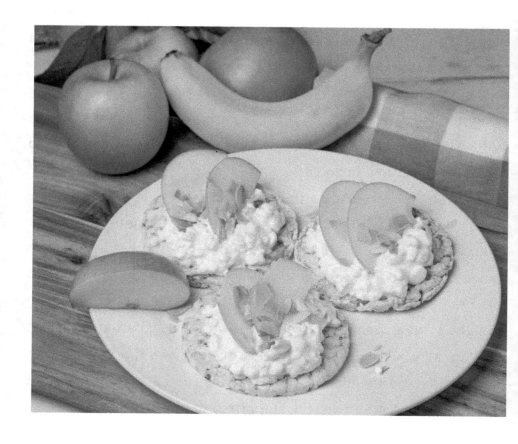

CHAPTER 1

FIRST OF ALL, WHAT IS A CHAFFLE?

These "Chaffles" are nothing more than waffles made with cheese. Hence the name "Chaffle" which derives from the union "Cheese" + "Waf- fle". People tied to the keto diet usually love chaffles. Grated cheese is a main ingredient in chaffle.

It's made with an egg and cheese batter instead of the flour-based batter you'll find in waffles. The high flour content in waffles adds a lot of carbohydrates, making them unhealthy according to the recommendations of the keto diet. Chaffles, on the other hand, have no flour. You can tell they're low-carb waffles with cheese.

The chaffles are extremely delicious. You won't realize that what you are actually eating is cheese eggs or cheese waffles. There are hundreds of chaffle recipes available, so you'll never miss out on options when you want to make one. There are also chaffles without cheese, for those who want to avoid or limit their intake of grated cheese.

CHAPTER 2

BENEFITS OF KETO DIET

The Keto diet has become so popular in recent years because of the success people have noticed. Not only have they lost weight, but scientific studies show that the Keto diet can help you improve your health in many others. As when starting any new diet or exercise routine, there may seem to be some disadvantages, so we will go over those for the Keto diet. But most people agree that the benefits outweigh the change period!

Benefits/Advantages

Losing weight: for most people, this is the foremost benefit of switching to Keto! Their previous diet method may have stalled for them, or they were noticing weight creeping back on. With Keto, studies have shown that people have been able to follow this diet and relay fewer hunger pangs and suppressed appetite while losing weight at the same time! You
are minimizing your carbohydrate intake, which means more occasional blood sugar spikes. Often, those fluctuations in
blood sugar levels make you feel hungrier and more prone to

snacking in between meals. Instead, by guiding the body towards ketosis, you are eating a more fulfilling diet of fat and protein and harnessing energy from ketone molecules instead of glucose. Studies show that low-carb diets effectively reduce visceral fat (the fat you commonly see around the abdomen increases as you become obese). This reduces your risk of obesity and improves your health in the long run.

Reduce the Risk of Type 2 Diabetes:

The problem with carbohydrates is how unstable they make blood sugar levels. This can be very dangerous for people who have diabetes or are pre-diabetic because of unbalanced blood sugar levels or family history. Keto is an excellent option because of the minimal intake of carbohydrates it requires. Instead, you are harnessing most of your calories from fat or protein, which will not cause blood sugar spikes and, ultimately, less pressured the pancreas to secrete insulin. Many studies have found that diabetes patients who followed the Keto diet lost more weight and eventually reduced their fasting glucose levels. This is monumental news for patients with unstable blood sugar levels or hopes to avoid or reduce their diabetes medication intake.

Improve cardiovascular risk symptoms to lower your chances of having heart disease:

Most people assume that following Keto is so high in fat content has to increase your risk of coronary heart disease or heart attack. But the research proves otherwise! Research shows that switching to Keto can lower your blood pressure, increase your HDL good cholesterol, and reduce your triglyceride fatty acid levels. That's because the fat you are consuming on Keto is healthy and high-quality fats, so they reverse many unhealthy symptoms of heart disease. They boost your "good" HDL cholesterol numbers and decrease your "bad" LDL cholesterol numbers. It also reduces the level of triglyceride fatty acids in the bloodstream. A top-level of these can lead to stroke, heart attack, or prema- ture death. And what are the top levels of fatty acids linked to?

High Consumption of Carbohydrates:

With the Keto diet, you are drastically cutting your intake of carbohydrates to improve fatty acid levels and improve other risk factors. A 2018 study on the Keto diet found that it can improve 22 out of 26 risk factors for cardiovascular heart disease! These factors can be critical to some people, especially those who have a history of heart disease in their family.

Increases the Body's Energy Levels:

Let's briefly compare the difference between the glucose molecules synthesized from a high carbohydrate intake versus
ketones produced on the Keto diet. The liver makes ketones
and use fat molecules you already stored.
This makes themmuch more energy-rich and an endless source of fuel compared to glucose, a simple sugar molecule. These ketones

can give you a burst of energy physically and mentally, allowing you to have greater focus, clarity, and attention to detail.

Decreases inflammation in the body:

Inflammation on its own is a natural response by the body's immune system, but when it becomes uncontrollable, it can lead to an array of health problems, some severe and some minor. The health concerns include acne, autoimmune conditions, arthritis, psoriasis, irritable bowel syndrome, and even acne and eczema. Often, removing sugars and carbohydrates from your diet can help patients of these diseases avoid flare-ups - and the delightful news is Keto does just that! A 2008 research study found that Keto decreased a blood marker linked to high inflammation in the body by nearly 40%. This is glorious news for people who may suffer from inflammatory disease and want to change their diet to improve.

Increases your mental Functioning Level:

As we elaborated earlier, the energy-rich ketones can boost the body's physical and mental levels of alertness. Research has shown that Keto is a much better energy source for the brain than simple sugar glucose molecules are. With nearly 75% of your diet coming from healthy fats, the brain's neural cells and mitochondria have a better source of energy to function at the highest level. Some studies have tested patients on the Keto diet and found they had higher cognitive functioning, better memory recall, and were less susceptible to memory loss. The Keto diet can even decrease the occurrence of migraines, which can be very detrimental to patients.

Decreases risk of diseases like Alzheimer's, Parkinson's, and epilepsy.

They created the Keto diet in the 1920s to combat epilepsy in children. From there, research has found that Keto can improve your cognitive functioning level and protect brain cells from injury or damage. This is very good to reduce the risk of neurodegenerative disease, which begins in the brain

because of neural cells mutating and functioning with damaged parts or lower than peak optimal functioning.

Studies have found that the following Keto can improve the mental functioning of patients who suffer from diseases like Alzheimer's or Parkinson's. These neurodegenerative diseases

sadly, have no cure, but the Keto diet could improve symptoms as they progress. Researchers believe that it's because of cutting out carbs from your diet, which reduces the

occurrence of blood sugar spikes that the body's neural cells have to keep adjusting to.

Keto can regulate hormones in women who have PCOS (polycystic ovary syndrome) and PMS (pre-menstrual syn- drome).

Women who have PCOS suffer from infertility, which can be very heartbreaking for young couples trying to start a family. For this condition, there is no known cure, but we believe it's related to many similar diabetic symptoms like obesity and a high level of insulin. This causes the body to produce more sex hormones, which can lead to infertility. The Keto diet paved its way as a popular way to regulate insulin and hormone levels and increase a woman's chances of getting pregnant.

Disadvantages

Your body will have a Changed period: It depends from person to person on the number of days that will be, but when you start any new diet or exercise routine, your body has to adjust to the new normal. With the Keto diet, you are drastically cutting your carbohydrates intake, so the body must adjust to that. You may feel slow, weak, exhausted, and like you are not thinking as quick or fast as you used to. It just means that your body is adjusting Keto, and once this change period is done, you will see the weight loss results you expected.

If you are an athlete, you may need more carbohydrates:

If you still want to try Keto as an athlete, you must talk to your nutritionist or trainer to see how the diet can be tweaked for you. Most athletes require a greater intake of carbs than the Keto diet requires, which means they may have to up their intake to ensure they have the energy for their training sessions. High endurance sports (like rugby or soccer) and heavy weightlifting requires more significant information on carbohy- drates. If you're an athlete wanting to follow Keto and gain the health benefits, it's crucial you first talk to your trainer before changing your diet.

You have to count your daily macros carefully:

For beginners, this can be tough, and even people already on Keto can become lazy about this. People are often used to eating what they want without worrying about just how many grams of protein or carbs it contains. With Keto, be meticulous about counting your intake to ensure you are maintaining the Keto breakdown (75% fat, 20% protein, ~5% carbs). The closer you stick to this, the better results you will see regard- ing weight loss and other health benefits. If your weight loss has stalled or you're not feeling as energetic as you hoped, it could be because your macros are off. Find a free calorie counting app that you look at the ingredients of everything you're eating and cooking.

CHAPTER 3

HOW TO MAKE THE PERFECT CHAFFLE

Here are some tips that will help you make fantastic chaffles

• Add a slice of chopped ham while mixing the egg and cheese. This will give you more protein and flavor. Those on a strict keto diet can also use bacon.

• Before adding the egg and cheese mixture, sprinkle some extra cheese on your waffle or chaffle maker. You will then have a savory and crispy chaffle.

• Don't open the waffle iron too early for checking. It should continue cooking until the chaffle is done and crisp. Let it cook for slightly longer for best results.

• Use mozzarella if you want your chaffle to be sweet. Cheddar cheese is good for savory chaffles. You can use Haloumi or goat cheese, but mozzarella is always the best
option because it is mild and not as greasy as many other
cheese varieties. Mozzarella will also reduce the eggy taste.

• Pepper jack cheese will give a slightly spicy taste. Almond/Coconut Flour in Chaffles

Chapter 4

SIMPLE CHAFFLE RECIPES

Chaffles With Raspberry Syrup

Servings: 4

Cooking Time: 38 Minutes

Ingredients:
- For the chaffles:
- 1 egg, beaten
- ½ cup finely shredded cheddar cheese
- 1 tsp almond flour
- 1 tsp sour cream
- For the raspberry syrup:
- 1 cup fresh raspberries
- ¼ cup swerve sugar
- ¼ cup water
- 1 tsp vanilla extract

Directions:

For the chaffles:

Preheat the waffle iron.

Meanwhile, in a medium bowl, mix the egg, cheddar cheese, almond flour, and sour cream.

Open the iron, pour in half of the mixture, cover, and cook until crispy, 7 minutes.

Remove the chaffle onto a plate and make another with the remaining batter.

For the raspberry syrup:

Meanwhile, add the raspberries, swerve sugar, water, and vanilla extract to a medium pot. Set over low heat and cook until the raspberries soften and sugar becomes syrupy. Occasionally stir while mashing the rasp- berries as you go. Turn the heat off when your desired consistency is achieved and set aside to cool.

Drizzle some syrup on the chaffles and enjoy when ready.

Nutrition Info:

Calories 105 | Fats 7.11g | Carbs 4.31g | Net Carbs 2.21g
Protein 5.83g

Cinnamon Powder Chaffles

Servings:2

Cooking Time: 5 Minutes

Ingredients:

- 1 large egg
- 3/4 cup cheddar cheese, shredded
- 2 tbsps. coconut flour
- 1/2 tbsps. coconut oil melted
- 1 tsp. stevia
- 1/2 tsp cinnamon powder
- 1/2 tsp vanilla extract
- 1/2 tsp psyllium husk powder
- 1/4 tsp baking powder

Directions:

Switch on your waffle maker.

Grease your waffle maker with cooking spray and heat up on medium heat.

In a mixing bowl, beat egg withcoconut flour, oil, stevia, cinnamon pow- der, vanilla, husk powder, and baking powder.

Once the egg is beaten well, add in cheeseand mix again.

Pour half of the waffle batter into the middle of your waffle iron and close the lid.

Cook chaffles for about 2-3 minutesutes until crispy.

Once chaffles are cooked, carefully remove them from the maker.

Serve with keto hot chocolate and enjoy!

Nutrition Info: Per Servings:

Protein: 25% | 62 kcal | Fat: 72% 175 kcal

Carbohydrates: 3% 7 kcal

Easy Chaffle With Keto Sausage Gravy

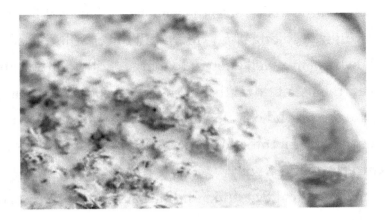

Serving: 2-3

Preparation Time: 5 Minutes

Ingredients

For Chaffle:

- 1 egg
- 1/2 cup of grated mozzarella cheese
- 1 Tsp of fine coconut flour
- 1 tsp of water
- 1/4 tsp of baking powder
- A Salt pinches
- For Keto Sausage Gravy:
- 1/4 cup of browned breakfast sausage
- 3 tbsp of chicken broth
- 2 tbsp of whipping cream, heavy
- 2 tsp of softened cream cheese
- garlic powder dash
- Add pepper to your taste
- dash onion powder (not mandatory)

Directions

Insert your Waffle Maker into the wall, as well as heat it up. Lightly grease or utilize cooking spray. Merge all the chaffle ingredients in a little bowl and mix well enough to merge. Add half the batter into the maker, then shut down the lid as well as cook for about 4 min

To prepare the second chaffle, Put the chaffle out from the waffle maker & do perform the same process. To be crispy, set aside

For Keto Sausage Gravy

Make one lb. of breakfast drain and sausage. For this, reserve one-fourth of a cup

Tip: From the leftover sausage, start making sausage patties as well as keep 1/4 of a cup for this dish to brown.

If you are unfamiliar with the sausage for breakfast, its crumble, such as ground beef.

Clean the extra oil from the pan and insert 1/4 cup golden brown break- fast sausage as well as the remaining ingredients, continues stirring to a boil.

Reduce the heat to medium, & continue cooking with the cover off to start thickening for about 5 to 7 min. If you want it to be very thick, you should apply some Xanthan Gum, though if you're careful with that as well, the gravy of keto sausage can thicken. Then as it cools, it would thicken much more.

1.Season with salt and pepper over the chaffles, to taste, and add a spoon- full of keto sausage gravy.

Nutritional Value:

212 kcal Calories | 17 g Fat | 3 g Carbs | 11 g Proteins

Nut-Free Keto Cinnamon Roll Chaffles

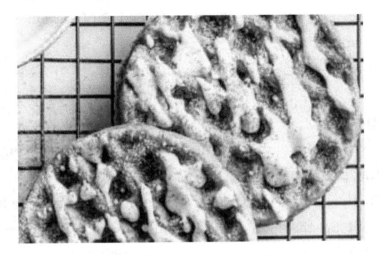

Serving: 2

Preparation Time: 15 min

Ingredients

For Batter:

- ½ cup of mozzarella cheese, shredded
- 2 tbsp of sweetener, golden monk fruit
- 2 tbsp of no-sugar-added "sun butter"
- 1 egg
- 1 tbsp of coconut flour
- 2 tsp of cinnamon
- ¼ tsp of vanilla extract
- ⅛ tsp of baking powder For Frosting:
- ¼ cup of powdered sweetener monk fruit
- 1 tbsp of cream cheese
- ¾ tbsp of melted butter

- ¼ tsp of vanilla extract or ⅛ tsp of maple extract
- 1 tbsp of coconut milk, unsweetened For Coating:
- 1 tsp of cinnamon
- 1 tsp of sweetener golden monk fruit

Directions

Switch on the waffle iron as well as enable to preheat during batter & frosting preparation

1.   Batter: Put all the batter's components together in a big mixing pot. Set the pot aside for 3-5 min to make the batter set Frosting: Mix over sweetener powdered monk fruit, sugar, maple or vanilla extract and cream cheese into a separate little combining bowl till smooth

Put in coconut milk then stir again till all components are well mixed.

Set it aside

Last steps: Brush preheated iron generously with non-stick cooking spray

Start dividing the chaffle mixture into 3 servings & spoon 1 portion into the waffle iron; when cooking, the batter spreads, leave a slight gap at the edges

Cook batter for around 2-4 minutes until the chaffle is lightly browned Open the lid of the waffle iron and allow the chaffle to cool down in the waffle iron for around 30 sec, before cautiously separating the chaffle, with a fork, at the edges and shifting it to a tray

Sprinkle cinnamon & monk fruit flavoring coating on chaffles when hot. Once mildly cools down, drizzle frosting atop chaffles

Notes:

•   Sun Butter replacement: If you do not have an allergy to the nuts, you could even replace in either (unsweetened) almond butter or (unsweetened) peanut butter besides Sun Butter at quite a 1:1 ratio.

•   Net Carbohydrates: One chaffle has 3.4 g of net carbohydrates in it.

•   Fridge Storage: In an airtight jar or freezing bag, place those keto chaffles inside the refrigerator & consume within 3 days.

•   Freezer Storage: In a freezing bag or airtight jar, place these chaffles and use a baking parchment sheet to divide each waffle so that they do not stick around each other. Place for 2 months in your freezer.

•   Reheating frozen or refrigerated chaffles: Use a toaster for reheating refrigerated chaffles, a preheated oven toaster, or a preheated microwave and heat until it is all cooked.

Nutritional Info:

195 kcal Calories | 15.1 g Fat | 31.5 g Carbs | 8.5 g Proteins

Garlic Chaffles

Servings:4

Cooking Time: 5 Minutes

Ingredients:

* 1/2 cup mozzarella cheese, shredded
* 1/3 cup cheddar cheese
* 1 large egg
* ½ tbsp. garlic powder
* 1/2 tsp Italian seasoning
* 1/4 tsp baking powder

Directions:

Switch on your waffle maker and lightly grease your waffle maker with a brush.

Beat the egg with garlic powder, Italian seasoning and baking powder in a small mixing bowl.

Add mozzarella cheese and cheddar cheese tothe egg mixture and mix well.

Pour half of the chaffles batter into the middle of your waffle iron and close the lid.

Cook chaffles for about 2-3 minutesutes until crispy.

Once cooked, remove chaffles from the maker. Sprinkle garlic powder on top and enjoy!

Nutrition Info: Per Servings:

Protein: 32% 36 kcal | Fat: 61% 69 kcal |

Carbohydrates: 7% 7 kcal

Spinach & Artichoke Chicken Chaffle

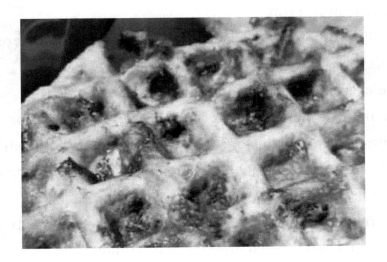

Servings: 2

Preparation Time: 3 minutes

Ingredients

- 1/3 cup of diced chicken, cooked
- 1/3 cup of cooked chopped spinach
- 1/3 cup of chopped marinated artichokes
- 1/3 cup of mozzarella cheese, shredded
- 1 oz of cream cheese, softened
- 1/4 tsp of garlic powder
- 1 egg

Directions

Preheat your waffle maker

Mix the garlic powder, eggs and cream cheese as well as Mozzarella cheese together in a little bowl

Add the chicken and artichoke and spinach and combine well

In your mini waffle maker, put 1/3 of the batter then cook it for four minutes. Let them cook for a further 2 minutes if they're still a little un- dercooked. Then cook the remaining mixture to create a second chaffle and finally prepare the final chaffle

Take it out from the maker after cooking and then let stay for two min Dip in sour cream, ranch dressing or celebrate alone

Nutritional Info:

172 kcal Calories | 13 g Fat | 3 g Carbs | 11 g Proteins

Zucchini Chaffles

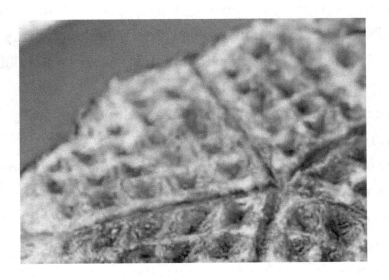

Servings: 2

Preparation time: 10 minutes

Ingredients

- 1 cup of grated zucchini
- 1 beaten egg
- 1/2 cup of parmesan cheese, shredded
- 1/4 cup of mozzarella cheese, shredded
- 1 tsp of dried basil, or maybe even 1/4 cup of chopped fresh basil,
- 3/4 tsp of divided Kosher salt
- 1/2 tsp of ground black pepper

Directions

Sprinkle on the zucchini approximately 1/4 teaspoon salt and then let it sit whilst collecting your ingredients. In a paper towel, wrap the zucchini before just using, then to force all the extra water out, squeeze it

Beat the egg in a little bowl. Combine the grated zucchini, basil, mozzarella, 1/2 tsp of salt, and pepper

Scatter 1-2 spoonful of chopped parmesan to coat the waffle iron base Scatter 1/4 of the mixture. Using about 1-2 tsp of chopped parmesan to cover and shut the lid. Using enough for surface covering. Check out the video and see how

Based on the size of the waffle maker cause the zucchini chaffle to be cooked for 4-8 mins. Usually, it is pretty much done when the processor has stopped the steam cloud emits. Let it cook till it's golden brown, for the great outcome

Remove it and repeat the same with the next waffle

Makes two full-size chaffles as well as four small chaffles, in the Mini maker

These chaffles freeze excellently. Freeze these, then warm them up again in the toaster or in your fryer to gain back crispiness.

Nutritional Info:

194 kcal Calories | 13 g Fat | 4 g Carbs | 16 g Proteins

Egg-free Coconut Flour Chaffles

Servings: 2

Cooking Time: 10 Minutes

Ingredients:

- 1 tablespoon flaxseed meal
- 2½ tablespoons water
- ¼ cup Mozzarella cheese, shredded
- 1 tablespoon cream cheese, softened
- 2 tablespoons coconut flour

Directions:

Preheat a waffle iron and then grease it.

In a bowl, place the flaxseed meal and water and mix well. Set aside for about 5 minutes or until thickened.

In the bowl of flaxseed mixture, add the remaining ingredients and mix until well combined.

Place half of the mixture into preheated waffle iron and cook for about 3-minutes or until golden brown.

Repeat with the remaining mixture. Serve warm.

Nutrition Info: Per Servings:

Calories: 76 | Net Carb: 2.3g | Fat: 4.2g Saturated

Fat: 2.1g | Carbohydrates: 6.3g | Dietary Fiber: 4g

Sugar: 0.1g | Protein: 3g

Easy Chaffle Sandwich

Servings: 1

Preparation time: 5 minutes

Ingredients
* 1 large egg
* 1/2 cup of mozzarella
* 1 tbsp (standard, gluten-free, almond or coconut flour)
* 1/2 tsp of baking powder
* 1 pinch salt

Directions
Coat nonstick cooking spray on the interior of a waffle maker. Preheat the waffle maker

Beat the egg in a little mixing bowl or cup. Mix the flour, baking powder, salt and combine properly

Stir in the scrambled cheese

Put the batter into the waffle iron. When using a mini-waffle machine, simply add in half of the mix

Lower with the cover. If the waffle maker has indicated the waffle is finished, raise the cover and transfer the waffle gently to a cooling rack. Use tongs to protect the fingertips from burning

Repeat this step until the amount of chaffles you want is reached

Nutritional Info:
269 kcal Calories | 17g Fat | 8g Carbs | 20 g Proteins

Cinnamon Roll Keto Chaffles

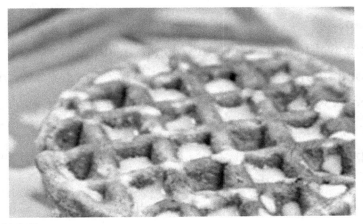

Servings: 1-3

Preparation Time: 5 minutes

Ingredients

- 1/2 cup of mozzarella cheese
- 1 tbsp of almond flour
- 1/4 tsp of baking powder
- 1 egg
- 1 tsp of cinnamon
- 1 tsp of Swerve, granulated
- For Cinnamon roll swirl
- 1 tbsp of butter
- 1 tsp of cinnamon
- 2 tsp of swerve
- For Cinnamon Roll Glaze
- 1 tbsp of butter
- 1 tbsp of cream cheese

- 1/4 tsp of vanilla extract
- 2 tsp of swerve

Directions

Insert your waffle maker into the plug to heat it up

Mix almond flour, mozzarella cheese, baking powder, 1 tsp of cinnamon as well as 1 tsp of granulated swerve and an egg in a small bowl, then set it aside

Add a tsp of cinnamon, 1 tbsp of butter, as well as 2 tsp of swerve sweet- ener to some other little bowl

Microwave it for 15 sec and combine well

Sprinkle the non-stick spray on the waffle maker, then pour 1/3 of the mixture to the maker. Float in 1/3 of the swerve, butter and cinnamon blend onto the upper part of it. Shut the maker and then let it cook for three or four minutes

When you complete making the first roll chaffle, start making the second one and after that, make the next

When the third chaffle is preparing, put 1 tbsp of butter in a medium bowl and 1 tbsp of cream cheese. Microwave it for 10 to 15 sec. Begin at 10, and when the cream cheese isn't really soft enough even to blend with the heat of butter, for an extra 5 seconds, heat it

Add the sweetener & vanilla extract to the cream cheese and butter, then combine well with a whisk

Drizzle on top of the chaffle with keto cream cheese glaze

Nutritional Info:

180 kcal Calories | 16 g Fat | 3 g Carbs | 7 g Proteins

Keto Oreo Chaffles

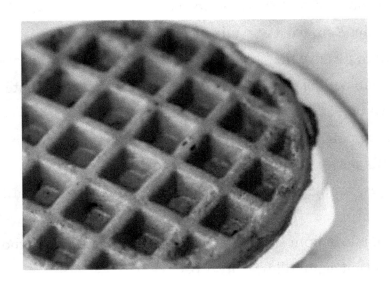

Servings: 2

Preparation Time: 15 min

Ingredients
- 1/2 cup of sugar-free Choco-chips
- 1/2 cup of butter
- 3 eggs
- 1/4 cup of Truvia, or even other sweeteners
- 1 tsp of vanilla extract
- Cream-Cheese Frosting
- 4 oz. of butter, at room temperature
- 4 oz. of cream cheese, at room temperature
- 1/2 cup of swerve, powdered
- 1/4 cup of whipping cream (heavy)
- 1 tsp of vanilla extract

Directions

Melt chocolate and butter in a protected bowl in a microwave for around 1 min. Remove it and mix nicely

You ought to just use the heat throughout chocolate and butter to melt the many of the chunks. You've over-cooked the chocolate whether you microwave till it's melted all over

Then get a spoon, as well as start to mix. If necessary, then add 10 sec, but mix perfectly before you intend to do so

Put the eggs, vanilla and sweetener in a bowl and combine until light & frothy

In a gradual flow, pour the melted chocolate and butter into the bowl, then beat again till well absorbed

Place approximately 1/4 of the blend into Mini Waffle Maker, then cook for 7-8 min or when it becomes crispy

Make the frosting as they cook

Put all the ingredients of frosting in a food processor's bowl and begin to process till fluffy and smooth. To achieve the right texture, you might need to put some more milk

To make the Oreo Chaffle, gently scatter or pipe the frosting amongst two chaffles

Should create 2 Oreo Chaffles in full size, or 4 Oreo Chaffles in mini size Tips

Just let waffles cool down more until they have eaten and frosting. It will enable them to be crispy.

To make the frosting, use the room temp butter and cream cheese.

Nutritional Info:

1381 kcal Calories | 146 g Fat | 14 g Carbs | 17 g Protein

Keto Caramelchaffle

Servings: 2

Preparation time: 10 Minutes

Ingredients

For the chaffles:

- 1 tbsp of Swerve sweetener
- 2 tbsp of almond flour
- 1 egg
- 1/2 tsp of vanilla extract
- 1⁄3 cup of mozzarella cheese, shredded for the caramel

sauce:

- 3 tbsp of unsalted butter
- 2 tbsp of swerve substitute of brown sugar
- 1/3 cups of whipping cream, heavy
- 1/2 tsp of vanilla extract

Directions

1. Let your waffle iron preheat

2. Put 3 tbsp butter as well as the 2 tbsp substitute of brown sugar together in a small pan or skillet over a moderate flame on the stove

3. Cook the sugar substitute blend and butter for 4 to 5 minutes till it starts to get brown (but not burn)

4. Insert the whipping cream in the blend, which is on the stove, as well as stir in very well. Cook the batter for ten minutes on a low boil before the mixture thickens and also has caramel sauce color

5. Mix all together components for the chaffles in a bowl, whereas the caramel sauce melts

6. Put half of the batter of the chaffle into the hot waffle maker then cook for 3 to 5 minutes till you have achieved the target degree of doneness

7. Take out the first chaffle, then cook the other half mixture for

another 3 to 5 min

8. Remove the final caramel sauce from the stove, and insert the vanilla extract. Let it cool a bit.

9. Put over the chaffles, the caramel sauce and eat

Nutritional Info:

189 kcal Calories | 18 g Fat | 2 g Carbs | 20 g Proteins

Dill Pickle Egg Salad Sandwiches

Servings: 2-3

Preparation time: 10 minutes

Ingredients

For egg salad:

- 6 eggs, hard-boiled
- ½ cup of dill pickles, chopped
- 3 tbsp of mayonnaise
- 1 tbsp of yellow mustard, prepared
- 1 tbsp of dill pickle juice
- 1 tbsp of dill, fresh
- Salt & pepper, as per your taste

For chaffles:

- 3 beaten eggs
- 1 tbsp of coconut flour
- 3/4 tsp of baking powder
- 1 1/2 cups of mozzarella finely chopped

Directions

To prepare egg salad:

Peel the eggs and chop them into tiny chunks

Put the eggs and remaining components to bowl. Mix well enough to combine

Eat right away or keep firmly wrapped in the refrigerator for up to four days

To prepare the chaffles:

Switch on to preheat your waffle maker

Stir the coconut flour, eggs as well as baking powder together. Add in the mozzarella cheese to integrate

Pour only enough mixture to cover the waffle iron bottom and shut the waffle iron. Cook them for 3 min. Take out the waffle and continue with the remaining mixture till you have prepared six chaffles

To assemble:

Split the egg salad equally among three chaffles Put the left chaffles on top of them and eat Notes

• If you would like to use almond flour instead of coconut flour, raise the quantity to 3 tbsp.

Nutritional Info:

465 kcal Calories | 35 g Fat | 7 g Carbs | 30 g Protein

Big Mac Chaffle

Servings: 2

Preparation time: 10 min

Ingredients

For cheeseburgers:

- 1/3 lb. of ground beef
- 1/2 tsp of garlic salt
- 2 pieces of American cheese

The Chaffles:

- 1 big egg
- 1/2 cup of mozzarella finely shredded
- 1/4 tsp of garlic salt For Big Mac Sauce:
- 2 tsp of mayonnaise
- 1 tsp of ketchup
- 1 tsp of dill pickle relish
- splash vinegar as per your taste to assemble:
- 2 tbsp of chopped lettuce
- 3 to 4 of dill pickles
- 2 tsp of finely chopped onion

Directions

Making the Burgers

Over a mid/high heat, heat the griddle

Split the beef into two spheres of similar size and put each, at about 6 inches away, on the griddle

Let them cook for around 1 minute

Using a tiny salad plate to push the beef balls tightly, to straight down to flatten. Scatter the garlic salt

Cook for 2 minutes, or when cooked half completely. Carefully turn the burgers, then spray lightly with the leftover garlic salt

Keep cooking for 2 min or till cooked completely

Put one cheese slice on each patty, then pile the patties onto a plate & set

aside. Wrap in foil to make the chaffles:

Heat and spray the waffle iron with non-stick cooking oil spray Mix the cheese, egg and garlic salt together until well mixed

In waffle iron, insert half egg mixture then cook for 2 to 3 minutes. Place aside and replicate the step with batter left over

Making Big Mac Sauce:

Mix all items together to organize burgers:

With stacked patties, chopped lettuce, onions, and pickle, top one chaffle Scatter the Big Mac sauce on the other chaffle, then put sauce on the sandwich face down

Eat right away

Nutritional Info:

831 kcal Calories | 56 g Fat | 8 g Carbs | 65 g Proteins

Keto Chaffle Garlic Cheesy Bread Sticks

Servings: 3-4

Preparation time: 3 Minutes

Ingredients

- 1 medium-sized egg
- 1/2 cup of grated mozzarella cheese
- 2 tbsp of almond flour
- 1/2 tsp of garlic powder
- 1/2 tsp of oregano
- 1/2 tsp of salt

For Topping

- 2 tbsp of unsalted softened butter
- 1/2 tsp of garlic powder
- 1/4 cup of grated mozzarella cheese

Directions

Turn the waffle maker on and grease it gently by using olive oil in a mixing bowl, whisk the egg

Insert the almond flour, mozzarella, oregano, garlic powder as well as salt and combine properly

Pour the mixture into the waffle maker Shut the cover and cook for about five min

Use tongs, pick the prepared waffles, then slice each waffle into 4 pieces Put these sticks on such a tray and heat the grill before that Combine the garlic powder and butter together and scatter on over sticks Spray the mozzarella over all the sticks and put for 2 to 3 min, under the grill till the cheese melts and make bubbles

Eat right away

Nutritional Info:

74 kcal Calories | 6.5 g Fat | 0.9 g Carbs | 3.4 g Proteins

Buffalo Hummus Beef Chaffles

Servings: 4

Cooking Time: 32 Minutes

Ingredients:

- 2 eggs
- 1 cup + ¼ cup finely grated cheddar cheese, divided
- 2 chopped fresh scallions
- Salt and freshly ground black pepper to taste
- 2 chicken breasts, cooked and diced
- ¼ cup buffalo sauce
- 3 tbsp low-carb hummus
- 2 celery stalks, chopped
- ¼ cup crumbled blue cheese for topping

Directions:

Preheat the waffle iron.

In a medium bowl, mix the eggs, 1 cup of the cheddar cheese, scallions, salt, and black pepper,

Open the iron and add a quarter of the mixture. Close and cook until crispy, 7 minutes.

Transfer the chaffle to a plate and make 3 more chaffles in the same manner.

Preheat the oven to 400 F and line a baking sheet with parchment paper. Set aside.

Cut the chaffles into quarters and arrange on the baking sheet.

In a medium bowl, mix the chicken with the buffalo sauce, hummus, and celery.

Spoon the chicken mixture onto each quarter of chaffles and top with the remaining cheddar cheese.

Place the baking sheet in the oven and bake until the cheese melts, 4 minutes.

Remove from the oven and top with the blue cheese. Serve afterward.

Nutrition Info:

Calories 552 | Fats 28.37g | Carbs 6.97g

Net Carbs 6.07g | Protein 59.8g

Basic Mozzarella Chaffles

Servings: 2

Cooking Time: 6 Minutes

Ingredients:

- 1 large organic egg, beaten
- ½ cup Mozzarella cheese, shredded finely

Directions:

Preheat a mini waffle iron and then grease it.

In a small bowl, place the egg and Mozzarella cheese and stir to combine. Place half of the mixture into preheated waffle iron and cook for about 2-minutes or until golden brown.

Repeat with the remaining mixture. Serve warm.

Nutrition Info:

Per Servings: Calories: 5 | Net Carb: 0.4g | Fat: 3.7g

Saturated Fat: 1.5g | Carbohydrates: 0.4g

Dietary Fiber: 0g | Sugar: 0.2g | Protein: 5.2g

Keto Chaffle Pizza

Servings: 2-3

Preparation time: 15-20 minutes Nutritional Info:

76 kcal Calories | 4.3 g Fat |

1.2 g Carbs | 5.5 g Proteins

Ingredients

- 1 egg
- 1/2 cup of crushed mozzarella cheese
- Only a pinch of seasoning, (Italian)
- 1 tbsp of pizza sauce (sugar-free)
- Topping with more crushed cheese pepperoni

Directions

Preheating the waffle machine

In the mixing bowl, beat the egg as well as seasonings together

Combine it with the crushed cheese and mix

To the hot waffle maker, insert a tablespoon of shredded cheese and then let it prepare for around 30 seconds. That will help produce a crisper crust

Apply half the batter to the machine then cook till it is golden brown & mildly crispy for around 4 min

To prepare the second chaffle, put the waffle out and insert the leftover mixture into the maker

Topping with pizza sauce, pepperoni and crushed cheese. Microwave it for around 20 seconds on high, and yes.

Basic Sweet Chaffles

Servings: 1

Preparation Time: 1 Minute

Ingredients

- 2 ounces of cream cheese
- 1 egg
- 1 tbsp of coconut flour
- 2 tsp of cocoa
- 1.5 tbsp of sweetener
- 1 tsp of vanilla
- 1/2 tsp of baking soda
- 1 tsp of cinnamon (not necessary)
- Oil Spray (Coconut)
- 1 tsp of butter (it's optional)

Directions

1.   For 20 seconds, put cream cheese in a microwave protected bowl then microwave it. (If cream cheese is already at room temperature, this step is not required)

2.   Add the remaining chaffle components with cream cheese into

the dish

3.   Socket-in and sprinkle your waffle iron with coconut oil

4.   Just put enough of your combined ingredients on the waffle machine

5.   Cover your maker, then patiently wait, yeah, that's going to be tough

6.   Remove the cooked chaffle and place it on a tray

7.   Top it with a butter slice

Nutritional Info:

230 Kcal Calories | 18 G Fat | 3 G Carbs | 23 G Proteins

Buffalo Chicken Chaffle

Servings: 2-3

Preparation time: 15 minutes

Ingredients

* ¼ cup of almond flour
* 1 tsp of baking powder
* 2 large eggs
* ½ cup of shredded chicken
* ¼ cup of mozzarella cheese, crushed
* ¼ cup of Frank's Red-Hot Sauce plus 1 tbsp (optional) for top- ping
* ¾ cup of shredded cheddar cheese, sharp
* ¼ cup of crushed feta cheese
* ¼ cup of diced celery

Directions

Mix and beat the baking powder into almond flour in a medium mixing bowl, then put aside

Preheat your waffle maker on mid/high heat, then brush with low-carb non-stick spray generously

Put the eggs in a mixing bowl and whisk till foamy Initially, insert in hot sauce & mix till well integrated Transfer flour batter to eggs and blend till all mixed

Lastly, put in crumbled cheeses then mix well till combined Mix in shredded chicken

Transfer chaffle mixture to preheated maker then cook till the outside browns. Approximately four minutes

Take it out from the waffle maker as well as perform step 7 till all the batter has been used up

Plate chaffles & it's top with celery, hot sauce or feta and serve

Nutritional Info:

675 kcal Calories | 52 g Fat | 8 g Carbs | 44 g Proteins

Keto Blt Avocado Chaffle Sandwich

Servings: 2-3 Preparation time:
20-30 minutes

Ingredients

- 3-4 bacon pieces
- 1 egg
- 1⁄2 cup mozzarella
- 1 tsp flour of almonds
- 1 tsp of all Bagel Seasoning (or preferably a sprinkle of salt, garlic, onion powder)
- 2 lettuce slices
- 1 sliced tomato
- 1 avocado slice
- 1 tbsp mayonnaise

Directions

For Bacon

Start with a cold saucepan. Put the bacon in the pan and turn on the heat to a minimum. At minimum temperature, bacon cooks better. When the bacon warms up a little bit and loses more of its fat, it begins curling up gently. You can then use tongs to rotate the bacon and start cooking on the other side.

Then proceed to turn consistently until all sides of the bacon are fried, around 10 minutes for thin or up to 15 minutes for thicker sliced bacon.

For Sandwich

Plugin, the Mini Waffle maker, to preheat

Crack the egg into a little bowl to create the chaffle and blend along with 1/2 cup mozzarella, almond flour and all bagel seasoning. This blend produces 2 chaffles

Pour 1/2 of the mix into the preheated chaffle maker and permit 3-4 min- utes of cooking (depending on how crispy you like your chaffles)

When cooking your first chaffle, prepare the tomato and avocado by cut- ting one slice of each

Pick up the chaffle and repeat for 3-4 minutes, adding the other half of the blend into the chaffle machine. When done, unplug the Waffle Machine In the chaffle, add your fried Bacon, then finish with lettuce, tomato, avocado and mayo

Put 2 toothpicks in the chaffle to tie them together and slice them in half. Your chaffle BLT avocado is ready to serve now

Nutritional Info:

208 kcal calories | 19.4g Fat | 3.1g Carbs | 20.3g Proteins

Chicken Quesadilla Chaffle

Servings: 1

Preparation time: 3 minutes

Ingredients

- 1/3 cup of cooked shredded chicken
- 1 egg
- 1/3 cup of cheddar jack cheese, shredded
- 1/4 tsp of taco seasoning, homemade

Directions

Preheat your waffle maker

Mix the taco seasoning and egg in a little bowl. When combined, add the cheddar cheese and the diced chicken

In the waffle maker, put 1/2 of the mixture then cook for four minutes. Let them cook for yet another two min if they're still a little uncooked. Then cook the leftover batter to create another chaffle

Dip in sour cream, salsa or savor alone

Nutritional Info:

135 kcal Calories | 10 g Fat | 1 g Carbs | 11 g Proteins

Hot Ham & Cheese Chaffles

Serving: 2-3

Preparation time: 5 minutes

Ingredients

- 1 large egg
- 1/2 cup of crushed swiss cheese
- 1/4 cup of deli ham, chopped
- 1/4 tsp of garlic salt
- 1 tbsp of mayonnaise
- 2 tsp of Dijon mustard

Directions

Plug it in to preheat the waffle iron

Beat the egg into a bowl. And add and combine in ham, cheese and garlic, salt

In the heated waffle iron, put half of the batter, cover it and cook for 3-4 min or till the waffle iron finishes steaming as well as the waffle is prepared completely

Transfer the waffle to a tray and continue with the batter leftover

Mix the mustard and mayo together to use as a sauce

Break the waffles into half or quarters then serve with sauce

Nutritional Info:

435 kcal Calories | 32 g Fat | 4 g Carbs | 31 g Proteins

Pumpkin Keto Chaffle Cake

Servings: 2

Preparation time: 10 min

Ingredients

For cake:

- 2 large eggs
- ¼ cup of pumpkin puree
- 2 tbsp of substitute brown sugar
- 2 tsp of pumpkin pie spice
- 2 tsp of coconut flour
- 1/2 tsp of vanilla
- 1 A cup of mozzarella cheese, finely shredded for frosting:
- 4 oz of cream cheese, at room temperature
- ¼ cup of butter, at room temperature
- ½ cup of sweetener, powdered
- 1 tsp of vanilla
- ¼ cup of crushed pecans

Directions

Plug-in, to preheat waffle machine. Sprinkle with non - stick cooking

spray

In a small bowl, add the pumpkin puree, eggs, sweetener and pumpkin pie spice, vanilla, coconut flour and stir well to mix

Mix in cheese

In the heated waffle iron, spoon one-fourth of the batter and spread the mixture out to the sides of the iron

Shut the iron and boil for 3 min

Take out and put aside the waffle. Repeat for batter left over Let the chaffles cool down before frosting

Beat butter and cream cheese together with an electronic mixer till soft and moist, to prepare the frosting. Stir till mixed well, the powder sweet- ener plus vanilla

Pour the frosting on the top of a chaffle and cover with another chaffle. Repeat layers and end with a frosting layer

Nutritional Info:

399 kcal Calories | 33 g Fat | 4 g Carbs | 11 g Proteins

Scatter with crushed pecans to beautify

Brie and Blackberry Chaffles

Servings: 4

Cooking Time: 36 Minutes

Ingredients:

- For the chaffles:
- 2 eggs, beaten
- 1 cup finely grated mozzarella cheese
- For the topping:
- 1 ½ cups blackberries
- 1 lemon, 1 tsp zest and 2 tbsp juice
- 1 tbsp erythritol
- 4 slices Brie cheese

Directions:

For the chaffles:

Preheat the waffle iron.

Meanwhile, in a medium bowl, mix the eggs and mozzarella cheese.

Open the iron, pour in a quarter of the mixture, cover, and cook until crispy, 7 minutes.

Remove the chaffle onto a plate and make 3 more with the remaining batter.

Plate and set aside. For the topping:

In a medium pot, add the blackberries, lemon zest, lemon juice, and erythritol. Cook until the blackberries break and the sauce thickens, 5 minutes. Turn the heat off.

Arrange the chaffles on the baking sheet and place two Brie cheese slices on each. Top with blackberry mixture and transfer the baking sheet to the oven.

Bake until the cheese melts, 2 to 3 minutes.

Remove from the oven, allow cooling and serve afterward.

Nutrition Info: Calories 576 | Fats 42.22g | Carbs 7.07g
Net Carbs 3.67g | Protein 42.35g

Turkey Chaffle Burger

Servings: 2

Cooking Time: 10 Minutes

Ingredients:

- 2 cups ground turkey
- Salt and pepper to taste
- 1 tablespoon olive oil
- 4 garlic chaffles
- 1 cup Romaine lettuce, chopped
- 1 tomato, sliced
- Mayonnaise
- Ketchup

Directions:

Combine ground turkey, salt and pepper. Form thick burger patties.

Add the olive oil to a pan over medium heat.

Cook the turkey burger until fully cooked on both sides. Spread mayo on the chaffle.

Top with the turkey burger, lettuce and tomato.

Squirt ketchup on top before topping with another chaffle.

Nutrition Info: Calories 555 | Total Fat 21.5g Saturated Fat 3.5g | Cholesterol 117mg | Sodium 654mg Total Carbohydrate 4.1g | Dietary Fiber 2.5g | Protein 31.7g Total Sugars 1g

Double Choco Chaffle

Servings: 2

Cooking Time: 10 Minutes

Ingredients:

*   1 egg
*   2 teaspoons coconut flour
*   2 tablespoons sweetener
*   1 tablespoon cocoa powder
*   ¼ teaspoon baking powder
*   1 oz. cream cheese
*   ½ teaspoon vanilla
*   1 tablespoon sugar-free chocolate chips

Directions:

Put all the ingredients in a large bowl. Mix well.

Pour half of the mixture into the waffle maker. Seal the device.

Cook for 4 minutes.

Uncover and transfer to a plate to cool.

Repeat the procedure to make the second chaffle.

Nutrition Info: Calories 171 | Total Fat 10.7g
Saturated Fat 5.3g | Cholesterol 97mg | Sodium 106mg Potassium
179mg | Total Carbohydrate 3g | Dietary Fiber 4 Protein 5.8g |
Total Sugars 0.4g

Cheddar Chicken & Broccoli Chaffle

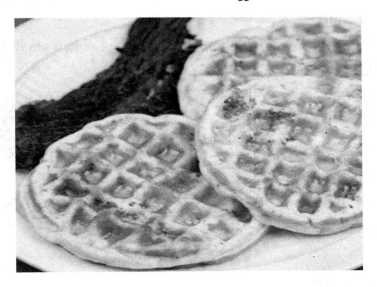

Servings: 2

Preparation time: 2 minutes

Ingredients

- 1/4 cup of diced cooked chicken
- 1/4 cup of chopped fresh broccoli
- Cheddar cheese, shredded
- 1 egg
- 1/4 tsp of garlic powder

Directions

Preheat your waffle maker

Combine the garlic powder, egg and cheddar cheese in a small bowl

Add the chicken & broccoli, then stir properly

In the waffle maker, put 1/2 of the batter then cook it for 4 min. Let them cook for a further 2 min if they're still a little uncooked. After this, cook the remaining mixture to prepare a second chaffle and finally cook the 3rd chaffle

Take it out from the pan after cooking and let it stay for two min Dip it in sour cream, ranch dressing, or you may enjoy alone

Nutritional Info:

58 kcal Calories| 1 g Fat | 1 g Carbs| 7 g Proteins

Keto Chaffles Benedict

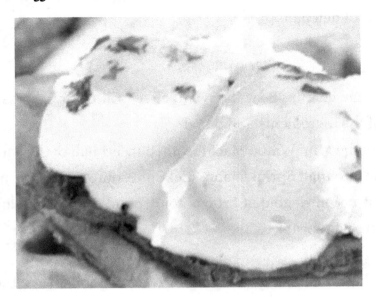

Servings: 2

Preparation time: 20 minutes

Ingredients

For Chaffle

- 2 egg whites
- 2 tbsp of almond flour
- 1 tbsp of sour cream
- 1/2 cup of mozzarella cheese For hollandaise
- 1/2 cup of butter, salted
- 4 yolks of eggs
- 2 tbsp of Lemon juice For poached eggs
- 2 whole eggs

- 1 tbsp of white vinegar
- 3 oz of deli ham4

Directions

Preparing the chaffle: Beat the white of egg till frothy, now add in the rest of the ingredients and blend

Preheating the Mini Waffle Machine, then insert half of the batter of the chaffle into that. Sprinkle non-stick spray onto the chaffle maker Cook till it becomes golden brown, for around 7 minutes. Pull the chaffle out and repeat

To make the Hollandaise sauce: organize a dual boiler (a pot which best fits on top with such a heat-safe bowl). Add sufficient water to boil in the pot, but do not contact the bowl's bottom

Hollandaise cont.: In the microwave, heat up the butter to boil. Place the egg yolks in the double boiler bowl and put the pot to boil. Transfer the heated butter into the bowl when boiling the pot

Hollandaise cont.: Beat nimbly heating the batter from the water under the bowl. Keep cooking till the pot water boils, the yolk-butter combination has thickened, as well as very extremely hot. Take the bowl out of the pot and insert the lemon juice. Set aside

To poach the egg: If required, add a little more water in the pot (you have sufficient to completely cover the egg) & take it to simmer. Put two tablespoons of white vinegar into the water. Drop an egg cautiously into the boiling water and cook it for 90 sec. Put it out using a slotted spoon to assemble: heat up the chaffle for some minutes in a toaster. Topping the crispy, crunchy chaffle with a poached egg, two tablespoons of hollandaise sauce and half of the ham pieces

Nutritional info:

352 kcal Calories | 26 g Fat | 4 g Carbs | 26 g Proteins

Cream Cheese Chaffle

Servings: 2

Cooking Time: 8 Minutes

Ingredients:

- 1 egg, beaten
- 1 oz. cream cheese
- ½ teaspoon vanilla
- 4 teaspoons sweetener
- ¼ teaspoon baking powder
- Cream cheese

Directions:

Preheat your waffle maker.

Add all the ingredients in a bowl. Mix well.

Pour half of the batter into the waffle maker.

Seal the device. Cook for 4 minutes.

Remove the chaffle from the waffle maker. Make the second one using the same steps.

Spread remaining cream cheese on top before serving.

Nutrition Info:

Calories 169 | Total Fat 14.3g | Saturated Fat 7.6g

Cholesterol 195mg | Sodium 147mg | Potassium 222mg

Total Carbohydrate 4g | Dietary Fiber 4g | Protein 7.7g

Total Sugars 0.7g

Keto Chaffle Blt Regular Sandwich

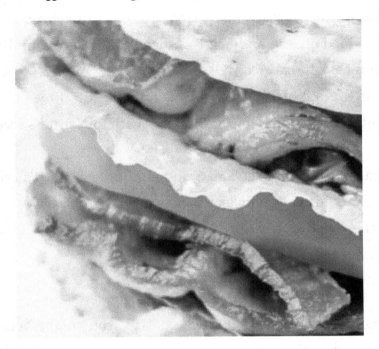

Servings: 2

Preparation time: 3 minutes

Ingredients

For chaffles

- 1 egg
- 1/2 cup of shredded cheddar cheese for sandwich
- 2 bacon strips
- 1-2 tomato slices
- 2–3 lettuce pieces
- 1 tbsp of mayonnaise

Directions

Preheat your waffle maker as instructed by the manufacturer

Mix the shredded cheese and egg together in a little mixing bowl. Mix until you have integrated well

Pour half of the mixture into the maker. Cook for three to four minutes, or till its light brown. Do the same with the batter's second half

Cook the bacon in a large saucepan on medium heat till it's crispy and switch as required. Remove onto paper towels to drain

Organize the sandwich with tomato, lettuce & mayonnaise. Celebrate it

Notes

If you're using a waffle maker of large size, you might become capable of cooking the entire batter amount in one waffle. That would vary with your machine's size.

Nutritional Info:

238kcal Calories | 18 g Fat | 2 g Carbs | 17 g Proteins

Keto Cauliflower Chaffles Recipe

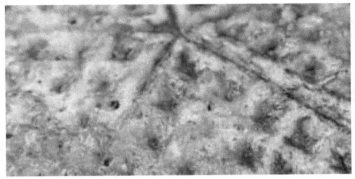

Servings: 1-2

Preparation time: 5 minutes

Ingredients

- 1 cup of cauliflower, riced
- 1/4 tsp of garlic powder
- 1/4 tsp of black pepper, ground
- 1/2 tsp of Italian Seasoning
- 1/4 tsp of Kosher salt
- 1/2 cup of mozzarella cheese shredded, or Mexican blend cheese shredded
- 1 egg
- 1/2 cup of parmesan cheese, shredded

Directions

Combine all the ingredients and put them into a blender

In waffle maker, scatter 1/8 cup of parmesan cheese. Ensure the waffle iron bottom is covered

Pour the cauliflower batter into the waffle machine

Put another scattering of parmesan cheese on the mixture's top. Ensure the top of the waffle iron is covered

Cook it for 4 to 5 min, or till its crispy

Tends to make four mini chaffles or two full-size chaffles

Nutritional Info:

246 kcal Calories | 16 g Fat | 7 g Carbs | 20 g Proteins

Keto Caramelchaffle

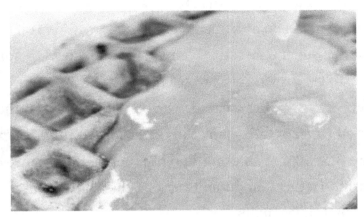

Servings: 2

Preparation time: 10 Minutes

Ingredients

For the chaffles:

- 1 tbsp of Swerve sweetener
- 2 tbsp of almond flour
- 1 egg
- 1/2 tsp of vanilla extract
- 1/3 cup of mozzarella cheese, shredded for

the caramel sauce:

- 3 tbsp of unsalted butter
- 2 tbsp of swerve substitute of brown sugar
- 1/3 cups of whipping cream, heavy
- 1/2 tsp of vanilla extract

Directions

1.   Let your waffle iron preheat

2.   Put 3 tbsp butter as well as the 2 tbsp substitute of brown sugar together in a small pan or skillet over a moderate flame on the stove

3.   Cook the sugar substitute blend and butter for 4 to 5 minutes till it starts to get brown (but not burn)

4.   Insert the whipping cream in the blend, which is on the stove, as well as stir in very well. Cook the batter for ten minutes on a low boil before the mixture thickens and also has caramel sauce color

5.   Mix all together components for the chaffles in a bowl, whereas the caramel sauce melts

6.   Put half of the batter of the chaffle into the hot waffle maker then cook for 3 to 5 minutes till you have achieved the target degree of doneness

7.   Take out the first chaffle, then cook the other half mixture for another 3 to 5 min

8.   Remove the final caramel sauce from the stove, and insert the vanilla extract. Let it cool a bit.

9.   Put over the chaffles, the caramel sauce and eat

Nutritional Info:

189 kcal Calories | 18 g Fat | 2 g Carbs | 20 g Proteins

Dill Pickle Egg Salad Sandwiches

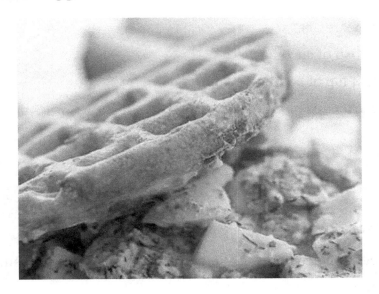

Servings: 2-3

Preparation time: 10 minutes

Ingredients

For egg salad:

- 6 eggs, hard-boiled
- ½ cup of dill pickles, chopped
- 3 tbsp of mayonnaise
- 1 tbsp of yellow mustard, prepared
- 1 tbsp of dill pickle juice
- 1 tbsp of dill, fresh
- Salt & pepper, as per your taste

For chaffles:

- 3 beaten eggs
- 1 tbsp of coconut flour
- 3/4 tsp of baking powder
- 1 1/2 cups of mozzarella finely chopped

Directions

To prepare egg salad:

Peel the eggs and chop them into tiny chunks

Put the eggs and remaining components to bowl. Mix well enough to combine

Eat right away or keep firmly wrapped in the refrigerator for up to four days

To prepare the chaffles:

Switch on to preheat your waffle maker

Stir the coconut flour, eggs as well as baking powder together. Add in the mozzarella cheese to integrate

Pour only enough mixture to cover the waffle iron bottom and shut the waffle iron. Cook them for 3 min. Take out the waffle and continue with the remaining mixture till you have prepared six chaffles

To assemble:

Split the egg salad equally among three chaffles

Put the left chaffles on top of them and eat Notes

- If you would like to use almond flour instead of coconut flour, raise the quantity to 3 tbsp.

Nutritional Info:

465 kcal Calories | 35 g Fat | 7 g Carbs | 30 g Protein

Cream Cheese Chaffle

Servings: 2

Cooking Time: 8 Minutes

Ingredients:

- 1 egg, beaten
- 1 oz. cream cheese
- ½ teaspoon vanilla
- 4 teaspoons sweetener
- ¼ teaspoon baking powder
- Cream cheese

Directions:

Preheat your waffle maker. Add all the ingredients in a bowl.

Mix well. Pour half of the batter into the waffle maker.

Seal the device. Cook for 4 minutes.

Remove the chaffle from the waffle maker. Make the second one using the same steps.

Spread remaining cream cheese on top before serving.

Nutrition Info:

Calories 169 | Total Fat 14.3g | Saturated Fat 7.6g Cholesterol 195 | mg Sodium 147mg | Potassium 222mg | Total Carbohydrate 4g Dietary Fiber 4g | Protein 7.7g | Total Sugars 0.7g

Big Mac Chaffle

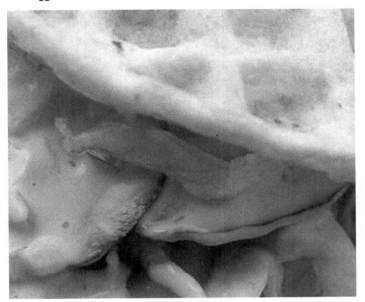

Servings: 2

Preparation time: 10 min

Ingredients

For cheeseburgers:

- 1/3 lb. of ground beef
- 1/2 tsp of garlic salt
- 2 pieces of American cheese

The Chaffles:

- 1 big egg
- 1/2 cup of mozzarella finely shredded
- 1/4 tsp of garlic salt For Big

Mac Sauce:

- 2 tsp of mayonnaise
- 1 tsp of ketchup
- 1 tsp of dill pickle relish
- splash vinegar as per your taste to assemble:
- 2 tbsp of chopped lettuce
- 3 to 4 of dill pickles
- 2 tsp of finely chopped onion

Directions

Making the Burgers

Over a mid/high heat, heat the griddle

Split the beef into two spheres of similar size and put each, at about 6 inches away, on the griddle

Let them cook for around 1 minute

Using a tiny salad plate to push the beef balls tightly, to straight down to flatten. Scatter the garlic salt

Cook for 2 minutes, or when cooked half completely. Carefully turn the burgers, then spray lightly with the leftover garlic salt

Keep cooking for 2 min or till cooked completely

Put one cheese slice on each patty, then pile the patties onto a plate & set aside. Wrap in foil

To make the chaffles:

Heat and spray the waffle iron with non-stick cooking oil

spray Mix the cheese, egg and garlic salt together until well mixed

In waffle iron, insert half egg mixture then cook for 2 to 3 minutes. Place aside and replicate the step with batter left over

Making Big Mac Sauce:

Mix all items together to organize burgers:

With stacked patties, chopped lettuce, onions, and pickle, top one chaffle Scatter the Big Mac sauce on the other chaffle, then put sauce on the sandwich face down

Eat right away

Nutritional Info:

831 kcal Calories | 56 g Fat | 8 g Carbs | 65 g Proteins

Egg-free Coconut Flour Chaffles

Servings: 2

Cooking Time: 10 Minutes

Ingredients:

- 1 tablespoon flaxseed meal
- 2½ tablespoons water
- ¼ cup Mozzarella cheese, shredded
- 1 tablespoon cream cheese, softened
- 2 tablespoons coconut flour

Directions:

Preheat a waffle iron and then grease it.

In a bowl, place the flaxseed meal and water and mix well. Set aside for about 5 minutes or until thickened.

In the bowl of flaxseed mixture, add the remaining ingredients and mix until well combined.

Place half of the mixture into preheated waffle iron and cook for about 3-minutes or until golden brown.

Repeat with the remaining mixture. Serve warm.

Nutrition Info: Per Servings:

Calories: 76 | Net Carb: 2.3g | Fat: 4.2g | Saturated Fat: 2.1g | Carbohydrates: 6.3g | Dietary Fiber: 4g | Sugar: 0.1g | Protein: 3g

Keto Chaffle Garlic Cheesy Bread Sticks

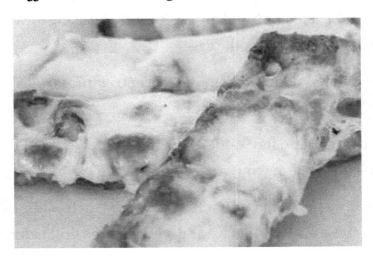

Servings: 3-4

Preparation time: 3 Minutes

Ingredients

- 1 medium-sized egg
- 1/2 cup of grated mozzarella cheese
- 2 tbsp of almond flour
- 1/2 tsp of garlic powder
- 1/2 tsp of oregano
- 1/2 tsp of salt

For Topping

- 2 tbsp of unsalted softened butter
- 1/2 tsp of garlic powder
- 1/4 cup of grated mozzarella cheese

Directions

Turn the waffle maker on and grease it gently by using olive oil in a mixing bowl, whisk the egg

Insert the almond flour, mozzarella, oregano, garlic powder as well as salt and combine properly

Pour the mixture into the waffle maker Shut the cover and cook for about five min

Use tongs, pick the prepared waffles, then slice each waffle into 4 pieces Put these sticks on such a tray and heat the grill before that

Combine the garlic powder and butter together and scatter on over sticks Spray the mozzarella over all the sticks and put for 2 to 3 min, under the grill till the cheese melts and make bubbles

Eat right away

Nutritional Info:

74 kcal Calories | 6.5 g Fat | 0.9 g Carbs | 3.4 g Proteins

Buffalo Hummus Beef Chaffles

Servings: 4

Cooking Time: 32 Minutes

Ingredients:

- 2 eggs
- 1 cup + ¼ cup finely grated cheddar cheese, divided
- 2 chopped fresh scallions
- Salt and freshly ground black pepper to taste
- 2 chicken breasts, cooked and diced
- ¼ cup buffalo sauce
- 3 tbsp low-carb hummus
- 2 celery stalks, chopped
- ¼ cup crumbled blue cheese for topping

Directions:

Preheat the waffle iron.

In a medium bowl, mix the eggs, 1 cup of the cheddar cheese, scallions, salt, and black pepper,

Open the iron and add a quarter of the mixture. Close and cook until crispy, 7 minutes.

Transfer the chaffle to a plate and make 3 more chaffles in the same manner.

Preheat the oven to 400 F and line a baking sheet with parchment paper. Set aside.

Cut the chaffles into quarters and arrange on the baking sheet.

In a medium bowl, mix the chicken with the buffalo sauce, hummus, and celery.

Spoon the chicken mixture onto each quarter of chaffles and top with the remaining cheddar cheese.

Place the baking sheet in the oven and bake until the cheese melts, 4 minutes.

Remove from the oven and top with the blue cheese.
Serve afterward.

Nutrition Info:

Calories 552 | Fats 28.37g | Carbs 6.97g | Net Carbs 6.07g

Protein 59.8g

Basic Sweet Chaffles

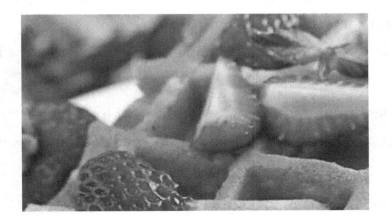

Servings: 1

Preparation Time: 1 Minute

Ingredients

- 2 ounces of cream cheese
- 1 egg
- 1 tbsp of coconut flour
- 2 tsp of cocoa
- 1.5 tbsp of sweetener
- 1 tsp of vanilla
- 1/2 tsp of baking soda
- 1 tsp of cinnamon (not necessary)
- Oil Spray (Coconut)
- 1 tsp of butter (it's optional)

Directions

1. For 20 seconds, put cream cheese in a microwave protected bowl then microwave it. (If cream cheese is already at room temperature, this step is not required)

2. Add the remaining chaffle components with cream cheese into the dish

3. Socket-in and sprinkle your waffle iron with coconut oil

4. Just put enough of your combined ingredients on the waffle machine

5. Cover your maker, then patiently wait, yeah, that's going to be tough

6. Remove the cooked chaffle and place it on a tray

7. Top it with a butter slice

Nutritional Info:

230 Kcal Calories | 18 G Fat | 3 G Carbs | 23 G Proteins

Buffalo Chicken Chaffle

Servings: 2-3

Preparation time: 15 minutes

Ingredients

- ¼ cup of almond flour
- 1 tsp of baking powder
- 2 large eggs
- ½ cup of shredded chicken
- ¼ cup of mozzarella cheese, crushed
- ¼ cup of Frank's Red-Hot Sauce plus 1 tbsp (optional) for top- ping
- ¾ cup of shredded cheddar cheese, sharp
- ¼ cup of crushed feta cheese
- ¼ cup of diced celery

Directions

Mix and beat the baking powder into almond flour in a medium mixing bowl, then put aside

Preheat your waffle maker on mid/high heat, then brush with low-carb non-stick spray generously

Put the eggs in a mixing bowl and whisk till foamy
Initially, insert in hot sauce & mix till well integrated
Transfer flour batter to eggs and blend till all mixed

Lastly, put in crumbled cheeses then mix well till combined
Mix in shredded chicken

Transfer chaffle mixture to preheated maker then cook till the outside browns. Approximately four minutes

Take it out from the waffle maker as well as perform step 7 till all the batter has been used up

Plate chaffles & it's top with celery, hot sauce or feta and serve

Nutritional Info:

675 kcal Calories | 52 g Fat | 8 g Carbs | 44 g Proteins

Keto Blt Avocado Chaffle Sandwich

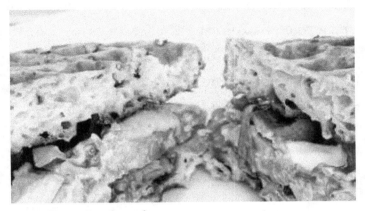

Servings: 2-3 Preparation time:

20-30 minutes

Ingredients

- 3-4 bacon pieces
- 1 egg
- ½ cup mozzarella
- 1 tsp flour of almonds
- 1 tsp of all Bagel Seasoning (or preferably a sprinkle of salt, garlic, onion powder)
- 2 lettuce slices
- 1 sliced tomato
- 1 avocado slice
- 1 tbsp mayonnaise

Directions

For Bacon

Start with a cold saucepan. Put the bacon in the pan and turn on the heat to a minimum. At minimum temperature, bacon cooks better. When the bacon warms up a little bit and loses more of its fat, it begins curling up gently. You can then use tongs to rotate the bacon and start cooking on the other side. Then proceed to turn consistently until all sides of the bacon are fried, around 10 minutes for thin or up to 15 minutes for thicker sliced bacon.

For Sandwich

Plugin, the Mini Waffle maker, to preheat

Crack the egg into a little bowl to create the chaffle and blend along with 1/2 cup mozzarella, almond flour and all bagel seasoning. This blend produces 2 chaffles

Pour 1/2 of the mix into the preheated chaffle maker and permit 3-4 min- utes of cooking (depending on how crispy you like your chaffles)

When cooking your first chaffle, prepare the tomato and avocado by cut- ting one slice of each

Pick up the chaffle and repeat for 3-4 minutes, adding the other half of the blend into the chaffle machine. When done, unplug the Waffle Machine In the chaffle, add your fried Bacon, then finish with lettuce, tomato, avocado and mayo

Put 2 toothpicks in the chaffle to tie them together and slice them in half. Your chaffle BLT avocado is ready to serve now

Nutritional Info:

208 kcal calories | 19.4g Fat | 3.1g Carbs | 20.3g Proteins

Keto Chaffle Pizza

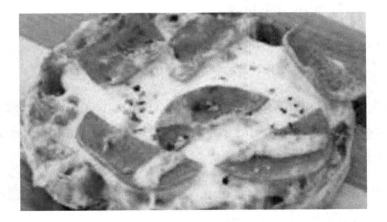

Servings: 2-3

Preparation time: 15-20 minutes

Ingredients

- 1 egg
- 1/2 cup of crushed mozzarella cheese
- Only a pinch of seasoning, (Italian)
- 1 tbsp of pizza sauce (sugar-free)
- Topping with more crushed cheese pepperoni

Directions

Preheating the waffle machine

In the mixing bowl, beat the egg as well as seasonings together Combine it with the crushed cheese and mix

To the hot waffle maker, insert a tablespoon of shredded cheese and then let it prepare for around 30 seconds. That will help produce a crisper crust

Apply half the batter to the machine then cook till it is golden brown & mildly crispy for around 4 min

To prepare the second chaffle, put the waffle out and insert the leftover mixture into the maker

Topping with pizza sauce, pepperoni and crushed cheese. Microwave it for around 20 seconds on high, and yes.

Nutritional Info:

76 kcal Calories | 4.3 g Fat | 1.2 g Carbs | 5.5 g Proteins

Chicken Quesadilla Chaffle

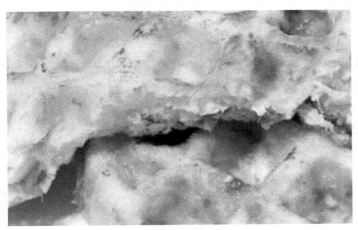

Servings: 1

Preparation time: 3 minutes

Ingredients

- 1/3 cup of cooked shredded chicken
- 1 egg
- 1/3 cup of cheddar jack cheese, shredded
- 1/4 tsp of taco seasoning, homemade

Directions

Preheat your waffle maker

Mix the taco seasoning and egg in a little bowl. When combined, add the cheddar cheese and the diced chicken

In the waffle maker, put 1/2 of the mixture then cook for four minutes. Let them cook for yet another two min if they're still a little uncooked. Then cook the leftover batter to create another chaffle

Dip in sour cream, salsa or savor alone

Nutritional Info:

135 kcal Calories | 10 g Fat | 1 g Carbs | 11 g Proteins

Basic Mozzarella Chaffles

Servings: 2

Cooking Time: 6 Minutes

Ingredients:

- 1 large organic egg, beaten
- ½ cup Mozzarella cheese, shredded finely

Directions:

Preheat a mini waffle iron and then grease it.

In a small bowl, place the egg and Mozzarella cheese and stir to combine. Place half of the mixture into preheated waffle iron and cook for about 2-minutes or until golden brown.

Repeat with the remaining mixture. Serve warm.

Nutrition Info: Per Servings:

Calories: 5 | Net Carb: 0.4g | Fat: 3.7g | Saturated Fat: 1.5g
Carbohydrates: 0.4g | Dietary Fiber: 0g | Sugar: 0.2g

Protein: 5.2g

Guacamole Chaffle Bites

Servings: 2

Cooking Time: 14 Minutes

Ingredients:

- 1 large turnip, cooked and mashed
- 2 bacon slices, cooked and finely chopped
- ½ cup finely grated Monterey Jack cheese
- 1 egg, beaten
- 1 cup guacamole for topping

Directions:

Preheat the waffle iron.

Mix all the ingredients except for the guacamole in a medium bowl. Open the iron and add half of the mixture. Close and cook for 4 minutes. Open the lid, flip the chaffle and cook further until golden brown and crispy, minutes.

Remove the chaffle onto a plate and make another in the same manner. Cut each chaffle into wedges, top with the guacamole and serve after- ward.

Nutrition Info: Per Servings:

Calories 311 | Fats 22.52g | Carbs 8.29g | Net Carbs 5.79g

Protein 13.g

Pumpkin Keto Chaffle Cake

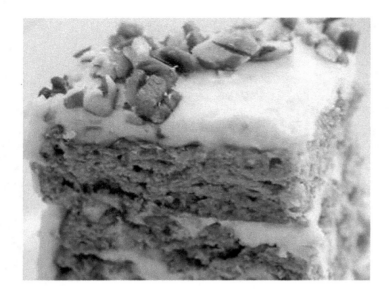

Servings: 2

Preparation time: 10 min

Ingredients For cake:

- 2 large eggs
- ¼ cup of pumpkin puree
- 2 tbsp of substitute brown sugar
- 2 tsp of pumpkin pie spice
- 2 tsp of coconut flour
- 1/2 tsp of vanilla
- 1 A cup of mozzarella cheese, finely shredded

for frosting:

- 4 oz of cream cheese, at room temperature
- ¼ cup of butter, at room temperature

- ½ cup of sweetener, powdered
- 1 tsp of vanilla
- ¼ cup of crushed pecans

Directions

Plug-in, to preheat waffle machine. Sprinkle with non - stick cooking, spray

In a small bowl, add the pumpkin puree, eggs, sweetener and pumpkin pie spice, vanilla, coconut flour and stir well to mix

Mix in cheese

In the heated waffle iron, spoon one-fourth of the batter and spread the mixture out to the sides of the iron

Shut the iron and boil for 3 min

Take out and put aside the waffle. Repeat for batter left over Let the chaffles cool down before frosting

Beat butter and cream cheese together with an electronic mixer till soft and moist, to prepare the frosting. Stir till mixed well, the powder sweet- ener plus vanilla

Pour the frosting on the top of a chaffle and cover with another chaffle. Repeat layers and end with a frosting layer

Scatter with crushed pecans to beautify

Nutritional Info:

399 kcal Calories | 33 g Fat | 4 g Carbs | 11 g Proteins

Brie and Blackberry Chaffles

Servings: 4

Cooking Time: 36 Minutes

Ingredients:

- For the chaffles:
- 2 eggs, beaten
- 1 cup finely grated mozzarella cheese
- For the topping:
- 1 ½ cups blackberries
- 1 lemon, 1 tsp zest and 2 tbsp juice
- 1 tbsp erythritol
- 4 slices Brie cheese

Directions:

For the chaffles:

Preheat the waffle iron.

Meanwhile, in a medium bowl, mix the eggs and mozzarella cheese. Open the iron, pour in a quarter of the mixture, cover, and cook until crispy, 7 minutes.

Remove the chaffle onto a plate and make 3 more with the remaining batter.

Plate and set aside. For the topping:

In a medium pot, add the blackberries, lemon zest, lemon juice, and erythritol. Cook until the blackberries break and the sauce thickens, 5 minutes. Turn the heat off.

Arrange the chaffles on the baking sheet and place two Brie cheese slices on each. Top with blackberry mixture and transfer the baking sheet to the oven.

Bake until the cheese melts, 2 to 3 minutes.

Remove from the oven, allow cooling and serve afterward.

Nutrition Info:

Calories 576 | Fats 42.22g | Carbs 7.07g | Net Carbs 3.67g

Protein 42.35g

Hot Ham & Cheese Chaffles

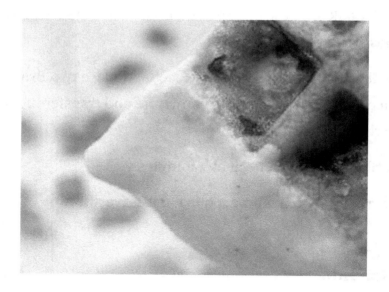

Serving: 2-3

Preparation time: 5 minutes

Ingredients

- 1 large egg
- 1/2 cup of crushed swiss cheese
- 1/4 cup of deli ham, chopped
- 1/4 tsp of garlic salt
- 1 tbsp of mayonnaise
- 2 tsp of Dijon mustard

Directions

Plug it in to preheat the waffle iron

Beat the egg into a bowl. And add and combine in ham, cheese and garlic

salt

In the heated waffle iron, put half of the batter, cover it and cook for 3-4 min or till the waffle iron finishes steaming as well as the waffle is prepared completely

Transfer the waffle to a tray and continue with the batter leftover Mix the mustard and mayo together to use as a sauce

Break the waffles into half or quarters then serve with sauce

Nutritional Info:

435 kcal Calories | 32 g Fat | 4 g Carbs | 31 g Proteins

Turkey Chaffle Burger

Servings: 2

Cooking Time: 10 Minutes

Ingredients:

- 2 cups ground turkey
- Salt and pepper to taste
- 1 tablespoon olive oil
- 4 garlic chaffles
- 1 cup Romaine lettuce, chopped
- 1 tomato, sliced
- Mayonnaise
- Ketchup

Directions:

Combine ground turkey, salt and pepper.

Form thick burger patties.

Add the olive oil to a pan over medium heat.

Cook the turkey burger until fully cooked on both sides.

Spread mayo on the chaffle.

Top with the turkey burger, lettuce and tomato.

Squirt ketchup on top before topping with another chaffle.

Nutrition Info: Calories 555 | Total Fat 21.5g | Saturated Fat 3.5g Cholesterol 117mg | Sodium 654mg | Total Carbohydrate 4.1g Dietary Fiber 2.5g | Protein 31.7g | Total Sugars 1g

Keto Pumpkin Chaffles

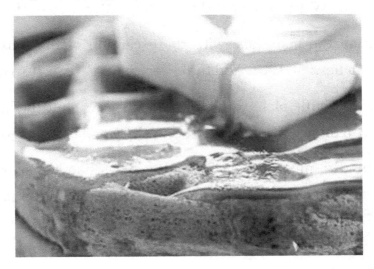

Servings: 2-3 Preparation Time: 2 min

Ingredients

- 1/2 cup of mozzarella cheese, shredded
- 1 egg beaten
- 1 1/2 tbsp of pumpkin purée
- 1/2 tsp of swerve
- 1/2 tsp of vanilla extract
- 1/4 tsp of pumpkin pie spice
- 1/8 tsp of maple extract, pure
- Optional: whip cream & sugar-free maple syrup, roasted pe- cans cinnamon, for topping

Directions

Switch on the Waffle Maker and begin the batter preparation

Insert in all the materials, with the exception of the mozzarella cheese, to a bowl and stir. Add the cheese in it and mix it so well

Sprinkle the waffle plate with a non-stick spray. Shut the lid, then cook for 4-6 mins depends on how crunchy you like the chaffles

Represent with any or some mix of toppings like butter, roasted pecans, sugar-free maple syrup, ground cinnamon dusting and a spoonful of whipped cream

NOTE

• You can also exclude this from the recipe if you do not have a pure maple extract, so they'll taste amazing!

Nutrition Values:

250 kcal Calories | 15 g Fat | 5 g Carbs | 23 g Proteins